Remote Medical Coding Jobs

60 Companies that hire Medical Coders

Shonda Miles,
MBA, CCS, CPC, CCS-P

www.remote-medical-coding-jobs.com

info@remote-medical-coding-jobs.com

To every new Medical Coding Student Graduate

You can do it!

Don't give up!

Contents

www.remote-medical-coding-jobs.com 2

Other books by Author 8

1. Thor Group 11

2. The CSI Companies *** 11

3. Nearterm 11

4. HIMagine (formerly Kforce) 11

5. Precyse 11

6. Harmony Health Staffing 11

7. Kindred Healthcare 12

8. Comforce 12

9. HC Tec Partners 12

10. National Staffing 12

11. Workbeast 12

12. Maxim Healthcare 12

13. UASI 13

14. Codebusters 13

15. Altegra Health 13

16. Cognisight 13

17. HCA Parallon 13

18. Hirschl& Associates 13

19. PCMS 14

20. RCM 14

21. Diskriter 14

22. Lexicode 14

23. Docucoders 14

24. TrustHSC *** 14

25. Signature Performance, Inc 15

26. MARSI 15

27. HIM Connections 15

28. HRS Solutions 15

29. Post Acute Medical 15

30. SVA MedCode Specialist 15

31. Amphion Medical Solutions 15

32. Aviacode *** 16

33. H.I.M. Recruiters 16

34. Greenville Health System 16

35. MDA Healthcare Consultants 16

36. Stern & Associates 16

37. Duke University Health System 17

38. The University of Mississippi Medical Center 17

39. 3M HIS 17

40. T-System 17

41. Amazon Coding 17

http://www.amazoncoding.com/#!apply/c1kns 17

42. Lenoir Memorial Hospital 17

43. North East Medical Services 17

44. ELAP Services, LLC 18

45. Optimum Healthcare IT 18

46. Coding Network 18

47. IOD 18

48. Piedmont Healthcare 18

49. Anthelio Healthcare Solutions 18

50. Banner Health 18

51. On Assignment HIM 19

52. Allied Health Group 19

53. Sutherland Global Services 19

54. CyberCoders 19

55. PopHealthCare 19

56. Peak Health Solutions 19

57. Panacea Health Solutions 20

58. Centra Health 20

59. Stanford Hospital & Clinics 20

60. Medpartners 20

61. Lakeshore Staffing & Recruiting 20

62. The University of Texas MD Anderson Cancer Center in Houston 21

63. Well Star Health 21

64. Future Net Technologies Corporation 21

65. Cooper Thomas LLC.. 21

66. Maine Medical Partners, MaineHealth 22

67. Kelsey-Seybold Clinic.. 22

68. DuvaSawko.. 22

69. JFK Medical Center.. 22

70. Centura Health 22

71 Metra 23

72. Rhode Island Hospital 23

73. Coders Direct.. 23

74. CIOX Health 23

75. Edgefield County Hospital.. 24

76. AGS Health 24

77. Holy Cross Hospital 24

78. Cooper Thomas, LLC *** 24

79. Adreima... 25

80. Froedtert Hospital*** 25

81. E-health jobs 25

82. ion Healthcare 25

83 25

84. Care National 26

85. The Coding Network, L.L.C 26

86. CEP America 26

87. GeBBS Healthcare 26

88. K.A. Recruiting 26

89 TTF 26

90. Excite Health Partners.. 26

90 Accounting Principals.. 27

91. Healthmedpharma 27

92. Practicemax... 27

93. Soliant Health 27

94. Insight Global *** 27

95. Para Health...27

96. Sterling Medical Corp..27

97. McKesson ***..27

98. Optum ***..28

99. Verisk ***...28

100. Inovalon ***...28

101. OS2Healthcare...28

102. Franciscan Alliance, Inc..28

www.remote-medical-coding-jobs.com..33

Excerpt from 18 Ways to Break into Medical Coding...34

Tip 1...34

Tip 2...34

Tip 3...35

Tip 4...36

Tip 5...36

Before You Leave...39

About the Author...40

Shonda Miles can be reached at www.remote-medical-coding-jobs.com or by email at info@remote-medical-coding-jobs.com...40

Other books by Author

10 Ways to Write an Ebook every 10 days

101 Success Questions

Remote Medical Coding Jobs

Tips for Staring an Online Business

How to Love Your Spouse again

How to Double Your Income in 12 Months or less

50 Tips to Jumpstart Your Success

50 Streams of Income

18 Ways to Break into Coding

How to Get the Job You want

21 Ways to Start a Marriage off Right

21 Ways to Make a Blended Family Work

AHIMA invites you to take part in the 2016 AHIMA Career Fair, October 18 and 19, 2016, to be held at the Baltimore Convention Center in Baltimore, MD. The AHIMA Career Fair is a must-attend for those seeking career advancement opportunities, professional development resources, and access to the industry's top employers.

http://careerassist.ahima.org/home/index.cfm?site_id=681

While I have made every attempt to make sure the information is accurate, there may be errors.

Also I have not listed any specific positions that may be available as I am sure you understand, this changes frequently.

"Allow yourself to dream and fantasize about your ideal life; what it would look like, and what it would feel like. Then do something every day to make it a reality!" Brian Tracy

"If you are willing to do more than you are paid to do, eventually you will be paid to do more than you do."

List of Remote Coding Companies

1. Thor Group

www.thorgroup.com

Send your resume to kathyw@thorgroup.com.

2. The CSI Companies ***

http://csihealthcareit.com/for-consultants/current-opportunities/

sbeatty@thecsicompanies.com

Send your resume to emrjobs@thecsicompanies.com

3. Nearterm

http://www.nearterm.com/category/him/

4. HIMagine (formerly Kforce)

http://blog.himaginesolutions.com/browse-jobs?_hstc=160187556.37cc5ff003f2567f373b46e8771252d2.1468864011274.1468864011274.1468864011274.1&_hssc=160187556.1.1468864011275&_hsfp=2838531800

5. Precyse

careers@precyse.com

Complete one page application at http://careers.precyse.com/search-our-job-listings/

6. Harmony Health Staffing

Complete Job Search Contact Form

http://harmonyhealthstaffing.com/findajob/jobsearchcontactform/

7. Kindred Healthcare

502-596-7898 FREE

Kindred Healthcare Support Center

8. Comforce

https://careers.acsicorp.com/

9. HC Tec Partners

http://hctec.com/careers/him-consulting/

Contact Information:
Deborah McNeese, HIM Recruiter
513-279-8304
dmcneese@hctec.com

10. National Staffing

http://nationalstaffhim.com/jobseekers/

http://www.nationalstaff.com/job-seekers/him.html

11. Workbeast

www.workbeast.com

http://workbeast.com/contact-us/

12. Maxim Healthcare

See more at:

https://www.maximhealthcare.com/careers/medical-coding-jobs.aspx

13. UASI

HR@uasisolutions.com

http://uasicoders.com/a-career-with-uasi-new/

Send your e-mail to HR@uasisolutions.com or visit: www.uasicoders.com

14. Codebusters

http://www.codebusters.com/jobs/

http://codingteams.codebusters.com/register.php

http://www.codebusters.com/medical-coders

15. Altegra Health

http://www.altegrahealth.com/careers/

16. Cognisight

http://www.cognisight.com/About/Careers

Please feel free to email your cover letter and resume to careers@cognisight.com.

17. HCA Parallon

http://www.parallon.com/careers

18. Hirschl& Associates

www.hirschl.net

Call (855) 236-0366 for openings

19. PCMS

mwright@pcms-consulting.com

http://www.pcms-consulting.com/

20. RCM

RCM Health Care Services

www.RCMHealthInformationManagement.com

http://www.rcmhealthinformationmanagement.com/career.html

21. Diskriter

Email your resume and information to:

careers@diskriter.com

http://www.diskriter.com/careers.html

22. Lexicode

https://www.talento.xyz/eFpWorkplace/logonInit.do?org=LEXICODE

Questions about employment can be emailed to us at careers@lexicode.com.

23. Docucoders

jobs@docucoders.com

http://docucoders.com/contact.php

24. TrustHSC ***

http://info.trusthcs.com/careers

25. Signature Performance, Inc

Suzanne Motta   smotta@signatureperformance.com

http://www.signatureperformance.com/Revenue-Cycle-Management/Medical-Career-Opportunities/positions.cfm?CFID=48991&CFTOKEN=75781350

26. MARSI

https://himexperts.com

lynn@himexperts.com

27. HIM Connections

http://www.himconnections.com/job-openings/

28. HRS Solutions

http://hrsolutions-inc.com/careers/#/jobs

29. Post Acute Medical

Jenny Navarijo   jnavarijo@warmsprings.org

http://www.postacutemedical.com/careers

https://careers-postacutemedical.icims.com/jobs/intro?hashed=-435768593&mobile=false&width=639&height=500&bga=true&needsRedirect=false&jan1offset=-360&jun1offset=-300

30. SVA MedCode Specialist

31. Amphion Medical Solutions

http://amphionmedical.mctesting.com

Amphion Medical Solutions
Attn: Stacey Haas, Coding Talent Specialist

888-830-2644

stacey.haas@amphionmedical.com
www.amphionmedical.com

http://amphionmedical.com/careers/#tab-id-2

32. Aviacode ***

Kris Cottrell   kris.cottrell@aviacode.com   http://www.aviacode.com

https://aviacode.catsone.com/careers/index.php?m=portal&a=listings&category=extraField196977&option=Medical+Coding+Jobs

33. H.I.M. Recruiters

Careers@HIMjobs.com

http://www.himjobs.com/search-jobs

34. Greenville Health System

http://www.ghscareers.org/

35. MDA Healthcare Consultants

http://www.mdahealthcareconsultants.com/employment.html

http://mdahealthcareconsultants.com/employment.html

36. Stern & Associates

http://www.stern-associates.com/

http://www.stern-associates.com/JobPostingsHIM.htm

37. Duke University Health System

https://www.hr.duke.edu/jobs/apply/index.php

38. The University of Mississippi Medical Center

39. 3M HIS

40. T-System

http://www.tsystem.com/careers

https://recruiting.ultipro.com/TSY1000/JobBoard/8a7c3806-d965-4081-16b8-11f42ca3055c

41. Amazon Coding

careers@amazoncoding.com

http://www.amazoncoding.com/#!apply/c1kns

42. Lenoir Memorial Hospital

Apply online at: www.lenoirmemorial.org.

43. North East Medical Services

http://www.nems.org

http://www.nems.org/careersPositions.html

44. ELAP Services, LLC

http://www.elapservicescareers.com/

45. Optimum Healthcare IT

http://www.optimumhit.com/contact-us

46. Coding Network

www.codingnetwork.com

http://www.codingnetwork.com/certified-medical-coder-jobs/

47. IOD

https://cioxhealth.jobs.net/en-US/join

48. Piedmont Healthcare

http://www.piedmont.org/PHC/careers-home.aspx

http://piedmonthealthcare.atsondemand.com/

49. Anthelio Healthcare Solutions

http://www.antheliohealth.com/career-notice.html

https://rn21.ultipro.com/PRO1004/JobBoard/ListJobs.aspx

50. Banner Health

Must live in 1 of the following states: AZ, CA, CO, IA, NE, NV, UT, WY

TameliaNorthnor via email at @ tamelia.northenor@bannerhealth.com

https://www.bannerhealth.com/careers

51. On Assignment HIM

http://www.oahim.com/job-seekers/apply

http://www.onassignment.com/careers-assignment

52. Allied Health Group

http://www.alliedhealth.com/cs/ccs-ahg/job-seekers

http://www.alliedhealth.com/job-seekers

Email **alliedhealthgroup@crosscountrystaffing.com**

53. Sutherland Global Services

http://www.sutherlandglobal.com/industries_healthcare_pr_Medical_Coding.aspx

http://www.sutherlandglobal.com/careers-SGS-Apply.aspx?ID=US

54. CyberCoders

Email your resume in Word to:
Sophia.Koo@CyberCoders.com
Sophia Koo - Executive Recruiter – CyberCoders

55. PopHealthCare

www.pophealthcare.com

http://www.pophealthcare.com/Careers

56. Peak Health Solutions

http://www.peakhs.com

https://careers-peakhs.icims.com/jobs/intro?hashed=-435771292&mobile=false&width=990&height=500&bga=true&needsRedirect=false

57. Panacea Health Solutions

http://panaceahealthsolutions.com/about-us/careers.html

58. Centra Health

In-patient/Out-patient Coding Analyst

https://www.centrahealth.com/careers

59. Stanford Hospital & Clinics

HIMS Inpatient / Outpatient Coders (Redwood City, CA or Remote)

Please direct all inquiries to Rosan Lam, Sr. Employment Specialist at RLam@stanfordmed.org. Submit your application online at www.stanfordhospitalcareers.com

60. Medpartners

http://www.medpartnershim.com/

http://www.medpartners.com/jobs/

61. Lakeshore Staffing & Recruiting

http://www.poweredbylakeshore.com

http://poweredbylakeshore.com/jobs/#s=1

62. The University of Texas MD Anderson Cancer Center in Houston

http://bit.ly/1U04xQu104629 Clinical Coding Specialist
http://bit.ly/1puu5c3104664 Mgr, Clinical Coding http://bit.ly/1R3CEaa

https://www.mdanderson.org/about-md-anderson/careers.html

63. Well Star Health

Wellstarcareers.org/jobs

http://www.wellstarcareers.org/index.asp

64. Future Net Technologies Corporation

Please copy and paste your resume in the body of e-mail and submit to hr@fnehr.com

https://www.web-cpr.com/onlineapply/

65. Cooper Thomas LLC

To apply, please go to the "Careers" section of our website at www.cooperthomas.com, and follow the instructions to register and apply.

http://cooperthomas.com/index.php/2014-01-22-19-03-51/postings

66. Maine Medical Partners, MaineHealth

Careersatmainehealth.org/locations/maine-medical-partners/

http://www.careersatmainehealth.org/

67. Kelsey-Seybold Clinic

http://www.kelsey-seybold.com/about-us/careers/pages/default.aspx

68. DuvaSawko

http://www.duvasawko.com/dscareers/

Email to hr@duvasawko.com

69. JFK Medical Center

JFK offers a highly competitive salary and benefits package reflective of our leadership position. Interested candidates are invited to send resume to Norma Merced at nmerced@jfkhealth.org. Please include cover letter along with resume and indicate CODE FROM HOME on the cover letter

 JFK Medical Center, 65 James Street, Edison, NJ 08820

70. Centura Health

www.centura.org/careers-and-education/

71 Metra

Email: jobs@metrarr.com - Full and Part Time Regular Job Opportunities ... *Please be sure to list the job title in the subject line of your email submission.

If you are interested in applying for a position at Metra, please send your cover letter which must include the position title*, and your resume to:

Email: jobs@metrarr.com - Full and Part Time Regular Job Opportunities
TempJobs@metrarr.com - Temporary and Intern Job Opportunities
http://www.lovelacehealthsystemjobs.com/?/work/job-post/outpatientcoderii106525

72. Rhode Island Hospital

https://www5.apply2jobs.com/Lifespan/ProfExt/index.cfm?fuseaction=mExternal.showSearchInterface

73. Coders Direct

CodersDirect.com opened their free job boards for both employers and coders on April 21, 2016.
I encourage you to consider posting your qualifications on CodersDirect.com to maximize your exposure to employers.
Mark Sluyter, Director, Member Services, Msluyter@CodersDirect.com

http://codersdirect.com/coder-registration/

74. CIOX Health

Contact: codingjobs@iodincorporated.com

For more information, visit www.CIOXHealth.com.

75. Edgefield County Hospital

Applications are available by printing directly from the Hospital web site at www.myech.org or by calling (803) 637-3174.

To be considered for the position, all interested persons should provide a completed application to:

Edgefield County Hospital
Attn: Nedra McRae
300 Ridge Medical Plaza
Edgefield, SC 29824

76. AGS Health

http://careers.agshealth.com/jobs/

77. Holy Cross Hospital

For immediate consideration, apply online at:
www.holy-cross.com/careers

78. Cooper Thomas, LLC ***

New coders welcome to apply

To apply, please go to the "Careers" section of our website at www.cooperthomas.com, and follow the instructions to register and apply.

79. Adreima

http://adreima.applicantstack.com/x/apply/a2r2jzxzmpod

80. Froedtert Hospital***

New coders welcome

https://careers.froedterthealth.org/ltm/CandidateSelfService/controller.se
rvlet?context.dataarea=ltm&webappname=CandidateSelfService&conte
xt.session.key.HROrganization=1000&context.session.key.JobBoard=F
H%20EXTERNAL&_saveKeys=true&JobPost=1&JobReq=9904&cont
ext.session.key.noheader=true#

81. E-health jobs

assist@e-healthjobs.com

Recruiter Name: Austin Morioka
Contact Phone: 808-258-2608

http://www.achcr.net/viewdetails.aspx?JobID=1175315&utm_source=In
deed&utm_medium=cpc&utm_campaign=Indeed

82. ion Healthcare

ionHealthcare provides training and equipment.

https://www.ionhealthcare.com/ionweb/Careers/index.cshtml

83. Beaufort Memorial Hospital

http://www.bmhsc.org/careers/job-openings/11895/content.aspx

84. Care National

http://carenational.com/career-opportunities/

85. The Coding Network, L.L.C

http://www.codingnetwork.com/certified-medical-coder-jobs/

86. CEP America

http://cepamerica.force.com/careers/ts2__JobSearch?nostate=1&f=a2wG0000000D1z8IAC&showJobs=500

87. GeBBS Healthcare

https://gebbs.com/about-us/careers/u-s-opportunities/

88. K.A. Recruiting

kristin@ka-recruiting.com

89 TTF

Interested and qualified candidates can send their resume to Chelle Bodnar at cbodnar@TTFrecruit.com.
- See more at:
http://jobs.cbizsoft.com/cbizjobs/jobs.aspx?cid=cbiz_ttr&consintid=&consid=&contactid=&source=#st hash.g96QoYPX.dpuf

Please send your resume to Kaitlyn at kzobel@ttfrecruit.com for consideration for Surgery Coders.
- See more at:
http://jobs.cbizsoft.com/cbizjobs/jobs.aspx?cid=cbiz_ttr&consintid=&consid=&contactid=&source=#st hash.g96QoYPX.dpuf

Interested and qualified candidates may send their resume to John Burns at jburns@TTFrecruit.com.
- See more at:
http://jobs.cbizsoft.com/cbizjobs/jobs.aspx?cid=cbiz_ttr&consintid=&consid=&contactid=&source=#st hash.g96QoYPX.dpuf

90. Excite Health Partners

http://excitehealthpartners.com/category/job/

90 Accounting Principals

http://www.accountingprincipals.com/JobSeekers/JobSearch/Pages/SearchResults.aspx?kws=coder&cty=&zip=&rds=50&submenuid=

91. Healthmedpharma

If you are interested in joining the HealthMedPharma team, please forward your resume to resumes@healthmedpharma.com

92. Practicemax

https://practicemax.applicantpool.com/jobs/

93. Soliant Health

Must live in Florida

http://www.soliant.com/jobs/search-results/

94. Insight Global ***

More Medical Coders Needed! 30 REMOTE openings. Can sit anywhere except California (due to OT and labor laws)... Start date is August 22... please send all resumes and questions to lcordell@insightglobal.net

95. Para Health

We are looking for a coder to do hospital facility coding. The position is remote and full time. Anyone interested can send their resume to mlehrer@para-HFCs.com.

96. Sterling Medical Corp

Position is for a medical coder at Wright-Patterson and a Medical Coding Trainer at Lackland Air Force Base and offers the following: Great Pay 2 Weeks Paid Time Off 10 Paid Federal Holidays Plus Benefits Hours are Mondays to Friday, 7:30am to 4:30pm Relocation Assistance Available if needed In addition to the above opportunity, we also offer various coding opportunities at select locations around the U.S. Emilie Munanga Recruiter/Staffing Coordinator Medical North America JV 411 Oak Street Cincinnati, OH 45219 Phone: (513) 984.1800 ext. 215 Toll Free: (800) 852.5678 ext. 215 Fax: (513) 984.4909 Email: emunanga@sterlingmedcorp.com

97. McKesson ***

https://careers.mckesson.com/

98. Optum ***

https://careers.unitedhealthgroup.com/search-jobs.aspx?kw=optum&lc=&jf=-1&inus=0

https://www.optum.com/about/careers.html

99. Verisk ***

http://careers.veriskhealth.com/

100. Inovalon ***

https://careers-inovalon.icims.com/jobs/intro?hashed=-435773209&mobile=false&width=580&height=500&bga=true&needsRedirect=false&jan1offset=-360&jun1offset=-300

101. OS2Healthcare

Website under construction

info@os2healthcaresolutions.com

http://os2healthcaresolutions.com/

102. Franciscan Alliance, Inc

http://www.franciscanalliance.org/careers/pages/default.aspx

Types of Medical Coding

Outpatient Pro Fee-Pro fee indicates a charge for the Physician. It means Professional.

Ambulatory Surgery (aka SDS same day surgery)-These surgeries are for a patient who is having surgery usually during the morning hours and goes home the same day. For the most part they go home unless there is an unexpected complication which might send them to observation.

Observation is when a patient is being observed for some condition. The doctor or the hospital can't justify an inpatient stay but they think the patient can benefit from being observed. Observation is considered Outpatient. There are two sets of observation Codes. 99218-99220 Initial Observation Services, where the patient is considered an outpatient. The facility does not need a designated observation area and patients are admitted to observation because their condition does not meet the status over a calendar day. 99217 is used for discharge from Observation Services. 99234-9936 is used for Observation Admission and Discharge Codes (same day). 992M 24-9226 is used for Subsequent Observation Services.

The CMS Claims Processing Manual (Medicare) describes: "For a physician to bill observation care codes, there must be a medical observation record for the patient which contains dated and timed physician's orders regarding the observation services the patient is to receive, nursing notes, and progress notes prepared by the physician while the patient received observation services. This record must be in addition to any record prepared as a result of an emergency department or outpatient clinic encounter."

For Medicare, same-day Observation services 99234-99236 require documentation of time in hours, with a minimum of eight hours documented. If duration of care is less than eight hours, then the 99218-99220 code set is appropriate. 99217 is not assigned when the patient is admitted and discharged from Observation during the same calendar date. If the patient is admitted and discharged on different days of services, Medicare does not require that the patient stay a minimum number of hours in order to bill for observation services.

Emergency Department (ED Coding) is services provided in the Emergency Department. Services provided are usually accidentally such as Poisonings, Accidents etc. You will also see nonemergency cases as well. Expect to code a lot of Accidents. This is considered an Outpatient Service. E/M levels typically include 99281-99285.

Interventional radiology Interventional Radiology is definitely something every coder should learn. It will make you more marketable. It will give you more confidence. You will always be high demand. Interventional Radiology Coders are among the highest paid. They tend to make $45-65 in most cases. While I don't have a certification in Interventional Radiology it certainly helps to build credibility and it will you do the job better. The procedures covered include Diagnostic angiography, non-vascular interventions, diagnostic cardiac catheterization and basic coronary arterial interventions and percutaneous vascular interventions.

HCC Hierarchical Condition Category is a payment model mandated by the Centers for Medicare and Medicaid Services (CMS) in 1997. This model is based on cumulative and chronic conditions. Basically an agency will come in and review a elderly patient's record for a year. The key is documentation here. The patient would have to be seen in that calendar year for the chronic conditions that they have for the doctor to get credit. Of course there is a lot more to this.

Ancillary Diagnosis Coding usually for Radiology tests. It is usually only the ICD-10-CM coding. This is the easiest type of coding for most. This is done usually for x-ray, drug, laboratory, or other services.

Outpatient Facility is Coding for Facility or the Hospital. It is Ambulatory Surgery Coding. It may include includes Injections and Infusions.

Inpatient Facility is inpatient coding for the hospital. There is a huge demand for inpatient coders. This is the hardest kind of coding next to Interventional Radiology. Also it is the second highest paid. This is any Procedures performed during the inpatient stay. The coder would code the diagnosis and procedures. The inpatient coder would review the entire record for the stay including the ER visit if there was one. Records tend to range from 8 pages to 300 pages depending on length of stay.

Inpatient Profee would be the Physicians portion of the hospital stay. Codes include 99221-99223.

This list is not exhaustive. It very well may vary from facility to facility. I hope this will give you an idea of how Medical Coding is broken down. This was meant to help you have a better understanding when you are speaking with HIM Professionals as well as Recruiters.

Acute care is usually referred to as inpatient care.

Level 1 Trauma is where your most severe inpatient care takes place. For example, Transplants, burn Unit etc,. You will tend to see longer hospital stays.

Level 2 Trauma is the next level. The cases here are not as severe.

How to make Six Figures as a Medical Coder

Are you a Medical Coder looking to make more money?

Do you want to earn at least $100,000 a year as a Medical Coder?

Are you tired of struggling as a Medical Coder?

Medical Coders are in big demand!

Don't miss the opportunity to get your share of the Medical Coding pie.

This webinar is for you if

- You are a medical Coder
- You want to become a medical Coder
- A seasoned medical coder
- Willing to work hard
- You like to read
- Goal oriented
- Ambitious
- Aggressive

This is not for you if are

- Lazy
- Looking for something quick and easy
- Have no interest in Medical Coding

In this 60-minute webinar you will Learn:

Top Four Paying Coding Areas

What you should be doing as a Coder

Know your worth

Five ways to earn $100,000 or more a year as a Medical Coder

Available on Demand

$99

www.remote-medical-coding-jobs.com

No fluff! Just action packed content for you to take action!

P.S. If you can't attend How to make Six Figures as a Medical Coder live, it will be recorded and you will receive the recording.

P.P.S. You don't want to miss this jam packed Webinar, you won't be sorry. This webinar will be recorded, you can view it anytime. You can watch it as many times as you like.

Excerpt from 18 Ways to Break into Medical Coding

Tip 1

Learn all you can while you're in school. In other words, I find students who rush through school just to try to finish so they can get a job. They just want to get through. They just want it done. This is totally understandable but this will be detrimental to their career.

To me this is a terrible thing to do because, while you can rush it and get through (the Medical Coding Program) and study enough to pass the test and make an A. This is horrible when it comes to actually working as a Medical Coder. You don't know medical terminology. You don't know key words that will help you do your job on a daily basis. You don't know why patients have XYZ.

It's so fundamental that you learn everything you can about Medical Terminology, Anatomy and Physiology, Disease process, drugs and lab tests. I speak from three points of view if you will. I have seen inpatient and outpatient coders struggle (I had to audit them), I've been an inpatient and an outpatient coder and I speak as someone who didn't learn myself. I see it as an instructor as well. I would have to say that inpatient is harder especially if you don't know these things.

For Outpatient Coders, you will need to know Medical Terminology and Anatomy and Physiology more so than the others. These other things if you knew them, disease processes, drugs, lab tests, they would be beneficial bonuses.

Tip 2

Good grades while you're in school will help you get a job. I get a lot of students that ask me for letters of recommendation- Maybe they haven't worked in a long time. Maybe their employer sent them to get this degree or finish this program so that they can transition from one job to another.

How does it look to ask for letters of recommendation and you made C's in the class? What can the instructor provide in a letter of recommendation for you?

Tip 3

The road for a coder is long and hard. I get a lot of students that tell me, that they want to do medical coding because they heard that it was easy. They can stay home. They can take care of their kids. They can do whatever they want and have a flexible schedule. This is a myth in a sense.

Yes, you can work from home, but you need to really bring your A game. You really need to be very knowledgeable about coding. You need to learn everything that you can so that when you're at home, you can figure things out. You have to have good research skills. You have to be able to figure things out on your own that maybe you don't know. So, it's not easy.

What I found is that I've worked remote for 6 years and people don't respect your time when you work from home. It could be a blessing and a curse. You find yourself really having a flexible schedule. You can do what you want and you tend to run around, do your errands during the day. Things that you would normally do after work, you can now do those during the day. You don't have to ask anybody if you want to go take your child to the doctor or if you want to go to the doctor.

It's a balancing act. It's not just being able to do what you want to. You still have to come back home and make up those hours.

Tip 4

Whenever you want to get a job as a medical coder, no matter if it's remote or not, you will have to pass a test. What I mean by "remote" is you work from home and maybe the hospital that you work for or, the recruitment company, maybe they're in another state. You still will have to take a test in order to get the job. A coding assessment is what they call it. You might receive a word document or a PDF file that you will have to complete. You have to pass the test in order to get the job.

Some companies have, an electronic version of the test. So, you would sign in to a secure website and you will get two hours or four hours to take the test approximately.

Tip 5

Be strategic if you want to get a job when you graduate from school. I advise all of my students to join the AAPC when they start going to school or at least go to all the meetings. Attend as a guest. I think it's $5 to attend as a guest. You can double check that at your local AAPC and that's at AAPC.com. You can see the local chapters, where they meet at, get on their list, or just start going as a visitor. Your school will probably have this information as well.

You can start going to meetings, networking, and find out who the people are that's there. I'm sure you'll find people there that are supervisors. You will find people that are already working in the field. The more you go, you start talking to people, building relationships, you'll be able to get a job once you graduate. For the first couple of meetings, just watch and observe. Of course, if someone ask you who you are be prepared to tell them.

If you're not sure about how to network, you want to read books about networking so you know how to build those relationships. You'll know how to stand out when an employer is looking for a new coder.

Do you know somebody that knows somebody? Who works for a doctor that could tell you if there's an opening, who could put a good word in for you.

I also, recommend that you actually go to the AHIMA local meeting. You can't actually do that unless you're a member of the National AHIMA. You could do that by going to AIHMA.org, and then becoming a member. You can select your local chapter at checkout for an $10. You can create a profile to receive alerts every single day about remote coding positions that they have available. You want to become active in the local chapter. You would do the same thing that you do for AAPC. You just want to meet the people that are there, become active. Of course, if you're a member of HIMAA as well as AAPC you can hold a position, you can do volunteer, you can learn as much as you can, then learn the people that are there.

Most people don't know as a medical coder that you have productivity standards, so you have to code so many charts per hour. Then you have accuracy standards as well, which means that maybe, you have to code 8 charts an hour and an accuracy rate of 95%. Some places it's a little bit more. You have to be 95% accurate on the charts that you code, so you really have to know your stuff, and be productive. Accuracy refers to how accurate the CPT codes and ICD-10 CM codes are.

For example, on the inpatient side it is somewhere between 3 or 4 charts per hour depending on length of stay. The production rate for Ambulatory Surgery charts, or Surgery charts is usually 6 to 8 charts per hour. These are the number of charts you would have to code and complete per hour. ED is a little bit more aggressive. If I'm not mistaken, it's somewhere around 20 charts per hour. More on this later.

These are strictly averages. This will vary from hospital to hospital.

If this was helpful you can purchase book from Amazon at

http://www.amazon.com/Ways-Break-into-Medical-Coding-ebook/dp/B01BW5EBZQ/ref=sr_1_1?ie=UTF8&qid=1462296543&sr=8-1&keywords=shonda+miles

Before You Leave

I need your help. When you go to the next page, Kindle gives you an opportunity to share your thoughts and opinions through your Facebook and Twitter account. If you believe your friends and family will benefit from this book, please share your thoughts with them. You might change someone's life, and I would be eternally grateful to you.

If you feel strongly about the contributions this book made to your life, please take a few seconds to post a 5-star review on Amazon. Very few people ever leave 5 star review. So it is a big deal if you do. Writing a 5-star review is like tipping me $25. I really appreciate the gesture. I feel like a million bucks whenever I get a glowing review.

If you have any questions, you can reach me via Shondamiles@yahoo.com. I will try to respond to your questions as soon as possible. You can also connect with me on Facebook and Twitter.

About the Author

Shonda Miles has been self-employed for 18 years. She has owned businesses ranging from an online retail store to a Training Company.

Shonda Miles is the CEO of Shonda Miles International, a company helping organizations and individuals improve performance and achieve their goals. Shonda Miles is here to help you achieve your full potential. Her purpose is to help millions of people achieve their goals and live their God given talent.

Shonda Miles is an Author, Entrepreneur, Speaker, Personal Development Trainer, Business Consultant and Business Coach. She loves reading Nonfiction books, writing business books and shopping. Personal Development is her mission. Shonda speaks, blogs and writes about a variety of personal development topics such as Time Management, Success, Goal Setting and having a Positive Attitude.

Shonda's goal is to help others achieve the level of success they desire.

Shonda Miles is a MBA Graduate. She has several successful businesses.

Shonda Miles can be reached at www.remote-medical-coding-jobs.com or by email at info@remote-medical-coding-jobs.com

Made in the USA
Middletown, DE
25 November 2016